The Alkaline Diet f[or kids]
Amazingly Delicio[us]
Recipes and Tips That Your Kids Will Love

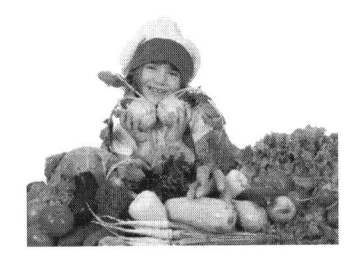

By Elena Garcia
Copyright Elena Garcia © 2014

Holistic Wellness Books

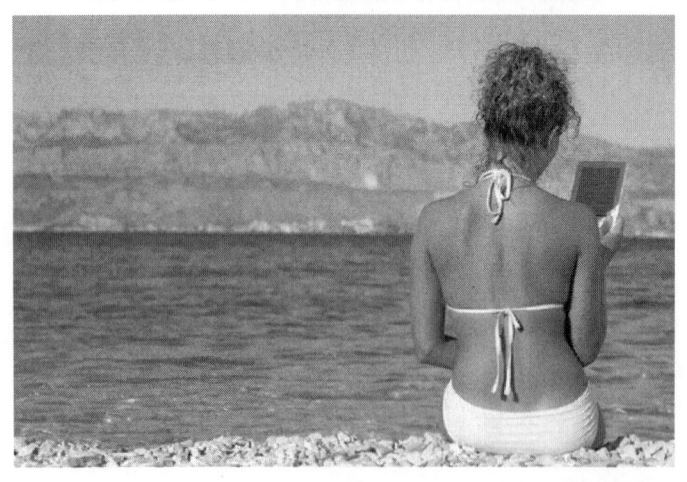

Visit and follow our page and be the first one to find out about new, hot releases as well as free and discounted eBooks dedicated to health, wellness and personal development:

www.facebook.com/HolisticWellnessBooks

www.twitter.com/Wellness_Books

All rights reserved. No part of this publication may be reproduced, stored in a retrieval system, or transmitted, in any form or by any means, electronic, mechanical, photocopying, recording or otherwise, without the prior written permission of the author and the publishers.

The scanning, uploading, and distribution of this book via the Internet or via any other means without the permission of the author is illegal and punishable by law. Please purchase only authorized electronic editions, and do not participate in or encourage electronic piracy of copyrighted materials.

Disclaimer:

A physician has not written the information in this book. It is advisable that you visit a qualified dietician so that you can obtain a highly personalized treatment for your case, especially if you want to lose weight effectively. This book is for <u>informational and educational purposes</u> only and is not intended for medical purposes. Please consult your physician before making any drastic changes to your diet.

TABLE OF CONTENTS:

ALKALINE DIET- INTRODUCTION...10

Benefits of an Alkaline Diet

My Personal Experience

ALKALINE TRICKS

THE ALKALINE DIET- BASIC CHARTS FOR BEGINNERS

ALKALIZING VEGETABLES

ALKALIZING FRUITS

ALKALIZING PROTEIN

ALKALIZING SWEETENERS

ALKALIZING SPICES & SEASONINGS

ALKALIZING OTHER

ACID VEGGIES AND FRUITS

ACID GRAINS

ACID BEANS/LEGUMES

ACID DAIRY

ACID NUTS

ACID ANIMAL MEATS AND ACID FATS

MORE ACID FOODS AND OTHER

ADDITIONAL HEALTHY ALKALINE TIPS FOR PARENTS

Chapter 1: Alkaline Breakfast Recipes…42

Recipe #1 Raspberry and Lemon Spread

Recipe#2 Banana and Chocolate Shake

Recipe#3 Bell Pepper Eggs

Recipe#4 Summertime Crazy Oats with a Twist!

Recipe#5 Winter Oats

    Recipe#6 Healthy Caffeine-free Kukicha Tea

    OPTION 1 KUKICHA CHAI TEA STYLE

    OPTION 2 KUKICHA VITAMIN C STYLE!

    OPTION 3 GRAPEFRUIT KUKICHA

    OPTION 4 ICE TEA SPA STYLE KUKICHA

    RECIPE #7 Alkaline Sandwich

RECIPE #8 Alkaline Paleo Mix: Bacon Spinach Eggs + Spanish Gazpacho Style Smoothie

RECIPE #9 Coconut Toasts

RECIPE #10 Raw Choco Spread Recipe

RECIPE #11 Raw Almond Butter Spread

Chapter 2: Alkaline Lunches...78

RECIPE #12 Brown Rice with Stir Fried Alkaline Vegetables

RECIPE #13 Creamy Mushroom soup with whole wheat garlic bread

Recipe#14 Tofu Salad Wrap

RECIPE #15 Yummy Salmon Salad

RECIPE #16 Mediterranean Pasta Salad with Tuna

RECIPE #17 Apple and Veggie Salad

RECIPE #18 Chicken Soup

RECIPE #19 Veggie Stir fry with Colors

RECIPE #20 Alkaline Vegetarian Curry

RECIPE #21 Sunday Veggie Roast Competition

RECIPE #22 Carrots Aperitif for Big Boys!

RECIPE #23Veggie Pizza

Chapter 3: Alkaline Afternoon/Evening Meals, Snacks and Dinners...108

RECIPE #24 Steamed Fish in Mint Paste and Lemon

Recipe #25 Whole Wheat Pasta with Tomatoes, Broccoli and Almonds

Recipe #26 Rose Flavored Soy Milk Pudding with Roasted Almonds on Top

Recipe #27 Capsicum and Corn Sandwich with Avocado Spread

Recipe #28 Spinach and Cottage Cheese Burger

Recipe #29 Quinoa and Coriander Stuffed Tomatoes

Recipe #30 Sweet Carrot Puree

Recipe #31 Sweet Apple and Cinnamon Drink

Recipe #32 Orange-Choco Smoothie

Recipe #33 Roibosh Banana Smoothie

Recipe #34 Mediterranean Fruit Salad

Recipe #35 Alkaline Spanish Granizado

Recipe #36 Apple-Kiwi Marmalade

Recipe #37 Wakame Energy Smoothie Made Sweet

Recipe #38 COCO Dream

Recipe #39 Delicious Apple Tortillas

Recipe #40 Kale and Spinach Chips

Recipe #41 Beet and Orange Magic!

Additional Tips...143

Conclusion...145

Alkaline Diet-Introduction

If you reside in the US, one look around and you will notice how obese our children have become. In fact, in the past 30 years, the number of obese children in the US has tripled. Almost 4 out of 10 kids are suffering from weight issues or obesity. The rest of the countries in the world are no different and are facing similar issues regarding obesity in children.

I visit my friends and relatives in Europe once or twice a year (Italy and Spain) and I am always petrified to notice how people go away from healthy and balanced nutritional patterns. Fast food is to blame! The way it is marketed, makes our children crave for it and some of them even detest healthy and nutritious food as a result!

Ever wondered how we got here? Well, let's analyze our lifestyles a bit. In our times, almost 20-30 years ago, children would often walk up to their school, played a lot of outdoor games and preferred an excursion trip over watching movies. There were no laptops, internet, gadgets and mobiles.

Food was usually eaten at home, eaten in smaller quantities and most importantly, it was full of nutrients and vitamins. Unlike today, the kids would eat porridge, leafy veggies or root vegetables which would help in the digestion process. There was less variety in supermarkets, as what was available was mostly real food. I also think that there were less distractions like the internet (not necessarily a bad thing, but if your kids spend all afternoons and evenings surfing the net, then I would say something should be done!).

It seems that even though our kids have unlimited access to all those movies and games, they still get bored. Too much of something can be a bad thing. I have observed this situation both in the US where I moved with my family as a teenager, as well as in Spain and Italy where I was born and lived as a kid (I am half Spanish, half Italian). What happens when our kids get bored? They feel like eating, but not because they are hungry, but because they are bored. Now, that I think about it, the same situation applies to us- adults! We set such a bad example sometimes!

Today, healthy food is replaced by pizzas, burgers, hot dogs and all kinds of starchy and junk items. This is one of the primary reasons we see obesity problems in kids from the age group of 6-12 years. In addition, lack of physical activities and indoor games has made our children lethargic.

What your kids eat plays an important role in maintaining their health and shaping their personality. No matter how cute those podgy little ones look, obesity can cause health issues like diabetes, tumors or even heart diseases in children. Not to mention their confidence; if you don't take care of their health, fitness and nutritional education now (me and my husband always say that these should be taught in schools!), you may make it extremely difficult for them when they become teenagers. They can feel insecure about their bodies and may not be successful as a result.

How can the Alkaline Diet help? I am sure that you have heard about it at least once. I would also like to ensure you that this is not another fad diet and that I have been practicing it faithfully for a few years now and so has my husband and our children. I also combine it with the Paleo Diet (my husband, James, loves Paleo!) and the Mediterranean Diet (my Southern European roots!). My first concern is to always make sure that we consume natural, unprocessed foods and eat at least 70% foods with alkalizing properties. Various studies have shown that alkaline diet could be the 'miracle food' that can reduce or completely cure obesity.

Alkaline diet

A human body needs a certain amount of acid and alkaline levels to maintain its pH balance. Acidic foods like whole flour, red meat or even too much fish can cause the acid levels in the body to shoot up and can completely throw the pH levels off balance. An alkaline diet focuses on consumption of leafy vegetables, whole grains and fresh fruits (less sugary ones) which help in preserving the pH balance.

Benefits of an Alkaline Diet

Let's have a look at how the alkaline diet can help in maintaining a child's health:

- **Helps in weight-loss**: Alkaline foods not only help maintain the pH balance in the body, but also help in battling obesity to a large extent. Since an alkaline diet contains a lot of dietary fiber, it helps in the digesting your food at a faster rate, thus improving your body's metabolism rate.

- **Makes the kid active**: Obesity can cause your child to not want to move around too much, adding to their problems. On the other hand, eating alkaline foods can help the body digest the food faster and act as a fuel for an active body.

- **Lesser Ailments**: Children who regularly consume alkaline foods in their daily diet suffer from fewer colds or flu. You don't need statistics to prove this. Mothers of obese children often complain about their kid's chronic illnesses or sudden flu. This is because acidic foods can lead to the development of harmful bacteria inside the body, thereby resulting in a weaker immune system.

- **Detoxifies the body**: Putting your child on the alkaline diet will ensure that the toxins from processed foods are flushed out easily. It can be used as a great detox diet which will maintain your child's health.

- **Focus and concentration**: Do you want your kids to do well with their studies? I do! This is why I have chosen the Alkaline Diet. I know that it helps them concentrate better, study faster and therefore enjoy the whole process of going to school, attending classes and learning new things. My boys also excel at sports and are always full of energy (which very often makes me and my husband less energetic as a result!).

My Personal Experience

My 7 year old son, Roberto, would often like to eat out at various food joints and restaurants. And like all other kids, he would sometimes relish a large pack of French fries or a hamburger on his way back from school. I became worried when this became a regular feature. He started skipping his meals as he would snack on some fried foods all the time, leaving no room for a proper meal. I may not be a doctor, but I guess being a mother is sometimes enough to know what's causing your child to have these health issues. I am sure that you, as a parent get the feeling!

Having been a victim of obesity myself as a child, I know how difficult life could get because of your weight issues. I have always been a "Chubby Kid" throughout my childhood and teens. I put on even more weight when my family and I moved to the United States. My mother would tell me stories about how "cute and cuddly" everybody found me, when in reality I was actually this fat little stout child. Little did she know about the way I was bullied in school.

For years I suffered a great amount of embarrassment and this escalated into my teenage years.

I thought getting into high school was a big sigh of relief as I would make new friends who would not care about how I look. This belief soon came crumbling down when I first entered my classroom and noticed some students talk about how big my arms look and how bulged out my stomach is.

At an age where I had imagined my life would get better, I was wallowing in self-pity. I realized that the only way I could help myself is by watching my food intake and the most importantly, the kind of foods I was consuming. I would read every little article about various diets and that's when I stumbled upon the benefits of alkaline foods, but I did not take action at first.

My experiences as a fat kid helped me become wiser about my food habits. I also made a promise to myself to pass on these good habits to my children so they could live a healthy life. In college, I decided to transform my body. I just made a decision to eat healthy and to exercise. I also did lots of research in nutrition and naturopathy.

Finally, I attended one of Tony Robbins's seminars (where I actually met my husband) and decided to explore the Alkaline Diet. Tony inspired me a lot (he always does!) and I knew that there was much more to this diet than just weight loss benefits. I understood that it was more like a lifestyle change and I was willing to do all it took to "make my life alkaline".

And so I did, and so did my husband!

But there were my sons who preferred nachos or acidic foods over an alkaline diet! Getting your kid to listen to you is quite a task. But isn't that always the case? Parenting is not easy after all. However, it's essential to understand the psyche of your kids. They are not going to want to do things just because you want them to.

Kids view healthy food as something 'sad'. So, I started whipping up a healthy dish in the most fun way. I also implemented a few strategies to make my dishes look more "Cool."

ALKALINE TRICKS

I am going to suggest a few tricks to get your kid to eat more fruits and vegetables.

- **Make the food look good**: Your kid is not going to want to eat your dish if it does not appeal to them. When you are cooking an alkaline rich meal for them, make sure that you are using different colored vegetables like red or yellow bell peppers, red or green apples or a yellow zucchini. Similarly, you can cut carrots or a pineapple in different shapes and use to decorate the dish. If necessary, use natural, raw honey, cinnamon or cocoa powder to make it sweet. Vanilla and stevia are also great and so is coconut milk.

- **Get them to participate**: I often ask my sons Roberto and Marco, to help me out while picking up groceries from the market. Make them feel that their suggestion matters to you and let them pick any one fruit or vegetable of their choice. This way your child will automatically get familiar with all kinds of healthy foods.

- **Let the food be fun**: The next time you bake a whole wheat bread for your kid, use a mould in the shape of a teddy bear or a famous cartoon and watch your child go gaga over it. This fun element in the food will ensure that your child looks forward to your next dish.

- **Reward them**: Each time they make the right food choice, appreciate them for their behavior. You can also reward them by letting them watch an extra episode of 'Pokemon' or play 'Angry birds'. However, you could also organize a nice day out, a picnic in a park with other kids, or a kids' party (with healthy foods of course). One thing is sure- you will have to learn how to make <u>creativity your friend</u>!

- **Let's draw**! Below are listed the rules of the alkaline diet and the basic charts for beginners. Do you know what we did to teach our sons which foods are good for them? A drawing game, yes! Just prepare 2, big pieces of colored paper. One is called "healthy alkaline foods", and the other one is called "unhealthy, acid foods". Write down different foods on small pieces of paper and mix them all up in a box. Tell your kids to close their eyes, pick up a word, read it, and tell you whether it's alkaline (healthy) or acidic (unhealthy). Score points and have fun!

  For example: look what I have here: "tasty and sweet carrot juice"- is it healthy or unhealthy?. Or: "A hot dog"- healthy on unhealthy?

  Then, you can also ask..."hmmm....but maybe we can make a healthy hot dog?" Go back to the list of unhealthy foods and meals and play another game- try to replace the ingredients and make it super healthy. This book will surely suggest how to do it.

This is a fantastic game that will help you spend more time with your loved **ones and have some fun!**

- **Crazy ice cubes!** This is a trick that I learned when visiting a good friend of mine in Spain. She taught me to mix water with fresh fruit juice as well as blueberries, raisins and other fruit pieces to make extremely creative ice cubes. Fruit ice cubes (you can even use beets) will give water an amazing color. You can also make fruit infused water and ask your kids to help you. Simply ask them: "hmm…I don't know how to make ice with all those fruits…I am sure that you know, can you help your mommy/daddy?"

- **Creative juices and smoothies- it's my turn game!**

Here is what we do- we always start a day with a nice smoothie or a juice. We have it before proper breakfast. We don't just live on smoothies, lol!

For example, Monday is my day. Tuesday is my husband's, Wednesday is Roberto's and Thursday is Marco's. Friday is a day when we pick up a weekly "juice contest winner "and there is always some celebration involved, Friday is our "have a nice meal out day" and so our winner chooses a nice place and gets treated there. We love discovering new restaurants in our town. We love vegan, vegetarian (we are not vegetarian, and I am not telling you to make your kids go vegan or vegetarian unless you want to, we just adore creative vegan and vegetarian food!), Thai, Japanese and of course Italian. When we go out we also get plenty of ideas for our weekend cooking. Yes! Every weekend we do massive cooking and we involve all 4 of us and we freeze the food for the rest of the week. Preparation and healthy means- no temptation later down the road.

THE ALKALINE DIET- BASIC CHARTS FOR BEGINNERS

Finally, I include the general overview of the Alkaline Diet.

Changing your diet to one that is full of alkaline foods is one of the easiest and best things you can do for your overall health. We were so ecstatic that we did! You should aim to intake 70/80 percent alkaline foods and 20/30 percent acidic foods. Once your pH is back on track, you can shift as we did to a 60 percent alkaline and 40 percent acid to maintain a high pH. Although, if you CAN stick to 80/20 then why not? We aim to eat this way most of the time.

For the most part, green veggies, many fruits, lentils, and seeds/nuts are considered alkaline.

While animals, their by-products, and all grains and legumes are acidic in general.

ALKALIZING VEGETABLES

-Alfalfa,

-Barley Grass,

-Beet,

-Broccoli,

-Cabbages,

-Carrot,

-Cauliflower,

-Celery,

-Chlorella (it's an alg),

-Cucumber,

-Dandelions,

- Dulce,

-Eggplant,

-Fermented Vegetables,

-Garlic,

-Greens,

-Green Beans,

 -Kale,

-Kohlrabi,

-Lettuces,

-Mushrooms,

-Mustard Greens,

-Nightshade Vegetables,

-Onions,

- Parsnips,

-Peas,

-Peppers,

-Pumpkin,

-Radishes,

-Rutabaga,

-Sea weed,

-Spirulina(it's an alg),

-Sprouts,

-Sweet Potato,

-Tomato,

-Watercress,

-Wheat-Grass

ALKALIZING FRUITS

-Apple,

-Apricot,

-Avocado,

-Berries (MOST),

-Cherry,

-Coconut,

-Currants,

-Date,

-Fig,

-Grape,

-Grapefruit,

- Lemon/Lime,

-Mango,

-Melon,

-Nectarine,

-Oranges,

-Peach,

-Pear,

-Pineapple,

-Raisin,

-Rhubarb,

-Tangerine,

-Tomato

ALKALIZING PROTEIN

-Almonds,

-Chestnuts,

-Millet,

-Fermented Tempeh,

-Fermented Tofu,

-Protein Powders (we love hemp)

ALKALIZING SWEETENERS

-Stevia,

-Agave,

-Maple

ALKALIZING SPICES & SEASONINGS

-Chili Peppers,

-Cinnamon,

-Curry,

-Ginger,

-Herbs,

-Miso,

-Mustard,

-Sea Salt,

-Tamari

ALKALIZING OTHER

-Alkaline Antioxidant Water,

-Apple Cider Vinegar,

-Bee Pollen,

-Fresh Fruit Juice,

-Fresh Vegetable Juices

ACID VEGGIES

-Olives, (what a shame! Elena loves them!)

-Winter Squash

ACID FRUITS

-Blueberries,

-Banana

-Canned fruit,

-Cranberries,

-Currants,

-Plums,

-Prunes.

ACID GRAINS

-Amaranth,

-Barley,

-Bran,

-Corn,

-Cornstarch,

-Flour (white, wheat, hemp),

-Kamut,

-Oats,

-Rice,

-Rye,

-Wheat

ACID BEANS/LEGUMES

-Black,

-Garbanzo,

-Kidney,

-Pinto, and White Beans,

- Lentils

<u>ACID DAIRY</u>

-ALL

ACID NUTS
-Cashew,

-Peanut,

-Pecan,

-Tahini,

-Walnut

ACID ANIMAL MEATS
-ALL

ACID FATS
-Canola,

-Corn,

-Flax,

-Hemp,

-Olive,

-Safflower,

-Sesame, and

-Sunflower Oils

MORE ACID FOODS AND OTHER ACID SWEETENERS

Carob, Corn Syrup, Sugar

ACID BEVERAGES
Alcohol, Coffee, Soda

ACID TOXINS AND DRUGS
All drugs, Weed killers, Insecticides, Tobacco

Now, there is debate on quite a few things as to whether or not they are alkalizing or acidifying. The good thing about the alkaline lifestyle is that we do not have to eat 100 percent alkaline. As long as we are taking in MOSTLY alkalizing foods, we are still on track! Here are some of the debated foods:

-Brazil Nuts,
-Banana (they are rich in magnesium which is an alkaline mineral, but they also contain lots of sugar which makes it acidic according to some charts).
-Brussels Sprouts,
-Buckwheat,
-Cashews,

-Chicken,

-Corn,

- Cottage Cheese,

-Eggs,

-Flax,

-Green Tea,

-Honey,

-Kombucha,

-Lima Beans,

-Non-dairy milks,

-Potatoes,

-Pepitas,

-Quinoa,

-Sauerkraut,

-Soy,

-Squash,

-Sunflower Seeds,

-Tomatoes,

-Yogurt.

I included many alkalizing and acidifying foods in this chapter, but of course, there are some that were not included. There are many different charts and lists available on the web. Sometimes, they may differ slightly but the most important thing to keep in mind is to choose just one of them and try to follow the alkaline way as much as possible. Remember- it's not only about eating 100% alkaline foods. Many charts include some acid-forming foods that are also considered healthy when consumed in moderation (e.g we love quinoa, oats, olives). Use charts as a guide, but don't worry too much if you find it difficult to memorize or if you have doubts whether your favorite food is alkaline enough. I always keep one of my 'alkaline charts' in my wallet at all times to reference at the grocery store.

ADDITIONAL HEALTHY ALKALINE TIPS FOR PARENTS

- You set an example for your children, you can't expect them to eat healthy, if your secret addiction is junk food. Trust me, they will know!
- Don't give them food (here I refer to unhealthy junk food) just because you want them to get busy or you wish to put them in a good mood. This is a really short-term solution and what can happen is that whenever they feel angry, sad or tired, they will just cry and ask you to get them this hamburger, pizza or kebab. Remember, you set an example and you have some responsibility to do!
- The more you cook at home and the more you get them involved- the better. Plus, you will also enjoy nice family time!
- Pizza, kebab, hot dogs- yes, but create your own, healthy and alkaline versions. Tofu is

great for that. You can also use gluten-free bread, wraps and pizzas. Remember to add plenty of green veggies.

It is my intention that this book helps you increase your creativity and also intuition when it comes to healthy cooking.

Healthy eating is FUN and your imagination is the only limit to what can be achieved.

Chapter 1: Alkaline Breakfast Recipes

Getting your kids to eat breakfast each morning before going to school can be difficult. Cooking a healthier and tasty breakfast for your child in so little time could be even more challenging. Breakfast is the most relevant meal of the day for your kid. For this reason, I am going to present you with the most instant and scintillating alkaline recipes.

Recipe #1 Raspberry and Lemon Spread

Kids just adore jams and spreads. Instead of buying them from the shops, you can make your own fresh fruit spread which is also alkaline in nature.

Ingredients

- 1 Big bowl of ripe raspberries
- 1/2 cup honey

- ½ teaspoon coconut oil

- Zest of about 2-3 lemons (so alkalizing!)

Preparation

1. Roughly cut the raspberries into small pieces and set them aside. Now, take some zest out of the lemons and sprinkle it on top of the raspberries.

2. Next, take a saucepan and place it on low heat. Add a teaspoon of coconut oil then the raspberries and the lemon zest. Let this mixture simmer for about 20-25 minutes on low heat until the raspberries turn into soft mushy lumps that can be smashed using a spoon.

3. Add a bit more honey to taste (optional, you can also use cinnamon) and cook it for another 10 minutes until the honey sugar gets dissolved completely. Now switch off the gas, add ½ a teaspoon of lemon juice and add ½ cup honey to it. Mix it well and let it cool down. You can store this

jam into an air-tight container and use it every morning.

Replacing sugar with raw, organic honey can help in increasing the nutritional value of the spread. I try to eliminate refined sugar to a minimum as it contains a considerable amount of empty calories.

Serving

This spread can be served with whole wheat bread, tortillas or can also be used a filling for whole wheat croissants. I always make my own bread and use a batman shaped mould for making this dish more exciting. If you are using readymade bread, you can use fun moulds to cut the bread into the shape of your child's favorite toon or superhero character. This is what we do! Our neighbors' kids loved the idea too!

Variations

- Instead of raspberries, you can also make use of pineapple, strawberries or even kiwi. Alternatively, you can use orange zest and orange juice in place of lemons. Use a different colored fruit each time you are out of spread.
- The same preparation with black grapes can taste even better.
- You can replace honey with ¾ cup of palm jiggery. This is only in case your child loves the taste of jiggery.

Recipe#2 Banana and Chocolate Shake (Serves 2)

Banana is rich in potassium which is extremely essential for growing kids. But to tell you the truth, I haven't come across too many kids who are fond of bananas. A banana chocolate shake not only tastes good but can also trick your kid to have bananas without knowing. Believe me, for days, my son, Roberto did not even know that the chocolate shake he adores had bananas and spinach in it.

Ingredients

- 1 ripe banana
- Half cup of baby spinach
- 400 ml chilled almond raw milk
- 2 teaspoon raw cocoa powder
- 2 drops of vanilla essence and cinnamon
- Optional: 1 tablespoon of flavored cornflakes for Garnish

Preparation

1. Roughly chop the banana and spinach, put it in a blender. Add the Cocoa powder.

2. Now, add ½ a teaspoon of honey or cinnamon and blend the mixture until it becomes a smooth paste. If the banana is completely ripe, you do not have to add sugar as the sweetness of banana is enough for the shake.

3. The next step is to add the chilled almond milk to it, also add two drops of vanilla essence. Blend it again for another 30 seconds. Check whether the shake is properly blended together and that there are no lump formations.

Serving

Take a tablespoon of flavored or unflavored cornflakes and crush them with your hand. Pour the milkshake in an attractive glass and sprinkle the crushed cornflakes on top of the shake for a nice crunch.

Variations

- Instead of banana, you can also use a ripe mango for this shake. But I wouldn't use mangoes too frequently as it's too sweet and could cause heat boils if consumed in excess.
- The cocoa powder used for this shake can be of any brand. I prefer Hershey as the Cocoa content in the powder is just perfect. Chocolate powder or dark chocolate can also make this shake yummier.
- If your kid does not like cornflakes, you can replace it with fruit loops or even cherries on top.
- Adding vanilla essence is optional. You can very well do without it.

Recipe#3 Bell Pepper Eggs (Serves 1-2)

Egg is one of the healthiest and protein rich foods to start your kid's day. The use of egg yolks however needs to be restricted, if you want to make it more alkaline, you can only use the egg whites.

Ingredients

- 2 or 3 Eggs
- Three slices of Bell Peppers (Red, yellow and green)
- 4 leaves of Spinach
- ½ teaspoon Pepper corn powder
- 1 teaspoon Himalaya salt
- Coconut oil

Preparation

1. Take fresh bell peppers, preferably of different colors and slice them into thin or thick rings depending upon how your kid likes it.

2. Now take a pan and grease it with some coconut oil. Heat the pan on slow heat for about 60 seconds. Place 3 slices of bell peppers on the pan with enough space in between each of them.

3. Break the eggs and pour them careful in the middle of each of those slices. Sprinkle some salt and pepper onto each piece.

4. Cover the pan with a lid for not more than 60-80 seconds. Just enough for the bell peppers to cook slightly. If you keep the pan covered for too long, it can cause the bell peppers to lose its color and there's also a risk of burning the eggs.

5. Switch off the gas and let the eggs sit on the pan for about 30 seconds or so. Carefully, take them out using a flat spatula and serve.

6. The next step is to chop the spinach into thin strips and deep fry them into hot oil on medium heat. When spinach is fried, it looks more attractive, is crunchier and also takes off the pungent taste that it's famous for.

Serving

Serve this dish preferably on a plain white dish. This works as a perfect background for the multicolored bell pepper eggs. You can either sprinkle the crunched spinach on top of each of these slices or serve it separately.

Variations

- If your child does not like bell peppers, you can use yellow or green zucchini.
- Spinach can be replaced with fried celery.
- Occasionally, you can use a circular cut-out of the whole wheat bread instead of bell peppers or zucchini.

Recipe#4 Summertime Crazy Oats with a Twist!

This recipe has a little surprise that is very refreshing!

Feel free to experiment with different fruits here. Since my sons love kiwis, and kiwis are a great source of vitamin C, we usually use them as a "special frozen ingredient"!

Ingredients (serves 2):

- 1 cup of Scottish oats (unprocessed)
- Half cup of raw almonds
- 1 tablespoon of cinnamon
- 2 cups of rice milk, or hazelnut milk, or almond milk
- 2 kiwis

- For the magic ice: 1 big avocado, 1 kiwi, 2 tablespoons of raw cocoa and 1 cup of almond milk

Instructions:

Before you go to bed don't forget to...:

1. Blend avocado and kiwi with cocoa powder and 1 cup of almond milk. Freeze into ice cubes that will be ready for next morning!

2. Soak oats and almonds in almond milk (or any other milk of your choice) and leave overnight.

   In the morning (so easy!):

   1. Mix oats with fresh kiwi slices and almond milk (can be also coconut milk or hazelnut milk).
   2. Add cinnamon.
   3. Add cocoa ice cubes!

Your kids will love this recipe, especially in the summer. My sons refer to it as "oats ice cream"!

Recipe#5 Winter Oats

This is a variation of the recipe#4.

In the winter, it's always better to start a day with something nice and warm.

Experiment with all kinds of alkaline friendly milks as: almond, rice and even coconut milk. We also like organic goat's milk from time to time.

Serves-2

Ingredients:

- 2 bananas
- A few raisins and almonds
- 1 cup of Scottish oats (unprocessed)
- 2 cups of your chosen vegan milk
- To garnish- blueberries or strawberries

Instructions:

1. Soak oats overnight

2. When you get up, simply mix all the ingredients and heat up until warm.

3. Add a few blueberries, strawberries or other fruit.

Recipe#6 Healthy Caffeine-free Kukicha Tea

My husband and I used to be caffeine addicts but we luckily managed to kick the habit. Now, we are addicted to all kinds of caffeine-free teas and infusions that our kids can also benefit from. This is an amazing alkaline drink that is suitable for kids and also for those who are caffeine-sensitive. Plus, we don't waste time preparing coffee for us and a separate drink for our boys. It's all in one solution. So practical!

There are different ways that you can prepare kukicha. We like to add a variety of tastes to our lives and our sons have turned out to be really creative as well. They always tell us to mix kukicha tea with different juices and vegan milk.

Kukicha tea can be also consumed chilled, and if you spice it up with ice, cinnamon and honey its taste will be amazing. Great for hot summers! Plus- no more artificial sweeteners and soft drinks. We are healthy, we are different and we are proud to inspire other families, this is what I always tell my kids and they love the idea.

OPTION 1 KUKICHA CHAI TEA STYLE

Serves-4, 5 cups

Ingredients:

- 1 liter of water
- 4 tea bags of kukicha tea
- 2 cups of almond milk
- 1 tablespoon of cinnamon

- 1 teaspoon nutmeg

- 1 tablespoon of grated ginger

- OPTIONAL: honey to make it sweet

Instructions:

1. Put water to boil.
2. Throw in kukicha tea bags. Stop the heat.
3. Add the spices and ginger and cover for a few minutes.
4. Add almond milk and stir.
5. Add some honey to sweeten if you want.
6. Serve warm or chilled with ice cubes, it's up to you!

OPTION 2 KUKICHA VITAMIN C STYLE!

Serves-4,5

Ingredients:

- 1 liter of water
- Juice of 2 lemons
- 2 tablespoons honey
- Optional: 1 glass of fresh apple juice

Instructions:

1. Put water to boil.
2. Add kukicha tea, turn the heat off.
3. Cover for a few minutes.
4. Add lemon juice and apple juice.
5. Sweeten with honey (you can also use natural stevia).
6. Serve warm or chilled with ice cubes.

OPTION 3 Grapefruit Kukicha

Grapefruits are alkalizing and so is kukicha tea. This is why they get on so well together!

Serves-4, 5 big cups

Ingredients:

- Juice of 4 big grapefruits
- 1 liter of water
- Kukicha tea, 4 tea bags
- Stevia to sweeten

Instructions:

1. Boil 1 liter of water.
2. Turn off the heat and throw in kukicha tea bags.
3. Cover and leave for a few minutes to brew.

4. Cool down a bit and add grapefruit juice and stevia to sweeten.

5. So alkaline and delicious!

OPTION 4 ICE TEA SPA STYLE KUKICHA

We love this recipe in the summer!

Serves-5

Ingredients:

- 1,5 liter of water
- 4 kukicha tea bags
- 2 limes, sliced
- 1 apple, sliced
- 1 banana, peeled and sliced
- 2 kiwis, peeled and sliced
- Ice cubes

Instructions:

1. Prepare the kukicha tea as in the previous recipes and let it cool down.

2. Pour cool kukicha tea in a big jar.

3. Add all the fruits and stir gently.

4. Cover and place in a fridge for 1 hour.

5. Add ice cubes and enjoy!

RECIPE #7 Alkaline Sandwich

Who said that bread is not allowed on an alkaline diet?

You can have good quality, gluten-free bread or wraps. Experiment with different varieties and choose your favorite bread!

We love to experiment with different kinds of alkaline sandwiches.

Now, I don't want you to think that I am trying to turn your kids into vegetarians (unless, of course, this is a lifestyle that you have chosen for your family).

This is why this sandwich has plenty of varieties. For example you can use avocado, or tuna, or sardines or even fried bacon. It's up to you. Of course, avocado is a super alkaline option. But, if you want, you can also mix it with some juicy bacon. My husband loves bacon and he is a big Paleo fan, this is why we try to mix different dietary approaches. Of course, we always remember to make at least 70% of our diet alkaline to keep healthy balance. Whenever buying meat, we choose organic. Local farmers are great for that.

Serves-1 (1 sandwich)

Ingredients:

- 2 slices of gluten free bread or wraps of your choice
- Olive oil or coconut oil
- Half cup of spinach
- Half avocado (peeled and sliced), or 1 can of tuna/sardines, or a few fried bacon strips (it's up to you!)
- A few big radishes, sliced
- 1 big tomato
- Half cucumber, peeled and sliced

- A few onion rings

- ¼ garlic clove, minced

- Black pepper

Instructions

1. Smear the bread with olive oil or coconut oil.

2. Spread avocado slices and if you want add tuna or bacon.

3. Add spinach, tomato, onion, cucumber, radish, a pinch of black pepper and garlic.

4. "Close" the sandwich or a wrap.

5. Serve with a few cucumber slices and parsley. So yummy!

RECIPE #8 Alkaline Paleo Mix: Bacon Spinach Eggs + Spanish Gazpacho Style Smoothie

Like I mentioned before, my husband is in love with Paleo! But he also loves Alkalinity.

This is a breakfast that all my 3 man absolutely adore and it also allows me to throw in some alkaline foods…find out how I do it!

Serves-3

Ingredients:

- 5 free range eggs
- A few bacon strips
- Coconut oil or olive oil
- 1 cup of baby spinach
- 2 garlic cloves

For Gazpacho style smoothie (super alkaline!):

- 8 ripe tomatoes (peeled),
- 4 cucumbers, peeled and chopped
- 1 onion, peeled and chopped
- 4 garlic cloves
- 1 cup of aloe vera or coconut water
- Juice of 1 lemon

Instructions:

1. Fry bacon in coconut or olive oil with 2 minced garlic cloves.
2. Add eggs and fry until done.
3. In a separate bowl mix baby spinach with olive oil and 2 garlic cloves (minced). Sprinkle over some lemon juice.

4. Prepare your plates. First, put spinach on each plate and then add bacon and eggs on top.

   Spinach, garlic and lemons are alkaline and so they will help you keep balance (bacon and eggs are of course acidic, but it's OK if you make them 30% of your diet and choose organic sources only).

5. Finally, blend all the ingredients for Spanish gazpacho style smoothie. So delicious and alkaline! Plus my men also get to enjoy their bacon and eggs!

6. Enjoy our Paleo Alkaline way and have a powerful day!

RECIPE #9 Coconut Toasts

The alkaline diet is about looking for healthy substitutes. I really recommend coconut oil as it is multifunctional. We don't even use butter anymore!

Now, everyone loves toasts in the mornings…It's just the smell that wakes you up!

Here is how we do it in our family.

Serves: 1 little toast

Ingredients:

- 1 slice of gluten-free bread of your choice, toasted
- 1 teaspoon of organic coconut oil
- Half avocado, sliced
- 1 lime
- A few cucumber slices
- Optional: fried bacon to add on top

- Himalaya salt
- Black Pepper

Instructions:

1. Toast the bread.
2. Smear your toast with some coconut oil.
3. Add avocado slices with cucumber.
4. Sprinkle over some fresh lime juice, Himalaya salt and pepper.
5. If you wish, add bacon on top. My men just love it!

RECIPE #10 Raw Choco Spread Recipe

Nutella is delicious and all kids love it! You can easily make your choco spread. It's healthier and cheaper.

Ingredients (for 1 cup of spread):

- 1 cup of almonds (soaked)
- A few tablespoons of raw cocoa powder
- Half cup of coconut milk
- 1-2 tablespoons of coconut oil for more consistency (optional).

Instructions:

1. Soak almonds in water or oats milk for at least a few hours.

2. In a blender, mix with coconut milk and blend until smooth. You may want to add more coconut milk, depends on your blender.

3. Add cocoa powder and stir energetically. Add coconut oil for more consistency.

4. Serve immediately, on a toast, or for better results, let it cool down in a fridge for a few hours.

MY TIP:

I use my choco spread to get my boys to eat more fruits. I learned this trick from my husband (Paleo, almost no bread style!). For example, you can slice apples, pears, grapefruits and peaches and use it as a toast- just smear it with some raw choco spread! Kids love it!

RECIPE #11 RAW ALMOND BUTTER SPREAD

Almonds are extremely alkaline and they can always be a great healthy spread ingredient for kids!

Ingredients (for 1 cup of a spread)

- Juice of 1 lemon
- 1 teaspoon of cinnamon powder
- 1 tablespoon of organic honey
- 1 cup of almonds, soaked
- Half cup of almond milk
- 1-2 tablespoons of coconut oil for more consistency

Instructions:

1. Soak almonds in water for at least a few hours.

2. In a blender, mix with almond milk, cinnamon, honey and lemon juice. Blend until smooth.

3. Experiment with coconut oil to achieve your desired consistency.

4. So yummy and alkaline!

Again, you can use it on bread, toast and sliced fruits. You can also mix it with smoothies and oat meals.

Chapter 2: Alkaline Lunches

When it comes to incorporating alkaline vegetables and fruits in your lunches, you can expect a highly tantalizing dish that will immediately catch your kid's attention. Between the breakfast and lunch, children lose a lot of energy trying to get ready for school, packing their bags or even trying to finish their last minute homework. For these reasons, the alkaline lunch is slightly heavier than the breakfast meals to provide them the right amount of energy for sustaining through the entire day.

RECIPE #12 Brown Rice with Stir Fried Alkaline Vegetables

(Serves 2 or 3)

There's nothing more sumptuous than a brown rice meal. Combine it with alkaline vegetables and you get the most energy filled lunch.

- 1 tablespoon olive oil
- 1 bowl of chopped Zucchini
- 1 bowl shredded cabbage
- 1 bowl of yellow, red and green bell peppers
- Two onions roughly sliced
- 3-4 Garlic cloves
- 1 bowl of carrots
- 1 tablespoon almonds
- 1 bowl of brown rice soaked in water for 15 minutes
- Salt to taste

Preparation

1. Chop zucchini, bell peppers, carrots and set them aside. Cut thin slices of garlic cloves.

2. Take a sauce pan and put one tablespoon of olive oil in it. Put it on slow heat and then add sliced garlic to it. 3.

3. When the garlic turns light brown, add onions and sauté for a while. Later add all the sliced vegetables and fry them for about 5 minutes on medium heat.

4. Now add the soaked brown rice, sprinkle some salt as per your taste and cover it with a lid. Let the rice cook for about 35-40 minutes on medium heat.

5. Brown rice typically takes longer to cook as compared to white rice. You may want to cook it for a little while longer if the rice does not seem cooked.

Serving

Serve in a colored plate and decorate it with a slice of pineapple on the side. To add some more crunch to it, you can use chopped parsley or spinach, deep fry it and sprinkle it on top of this dish. Alternatively you can always add fresh cherries to the rice.

Variations

- You can replace zucchini or bell peppers with any other alkaline vegetables.
- If you don't have soy sauce, you can do without it.
- You can swap the pineapple and use green apples instead. Nevertheless, pineapple tastes a lot better.
- You can either add uncooked brown rice to the vegetables or cook it together or you can add boiled rice and fry it with the vegetables for 3-4 minutes.
- Like all kids, if your kid loves noodles too, you can use boiled wheat noodles instead of rice in this recipe.

RECIPE #13 Creamy Mushroom soup with whole wheat garlic bread (serves 2)

Mushrooms are not only super tasty, but are also a great source of Vitamin D. Adding a bit of cream can get you a creamy texture and make it all the more delicious.

Ingredients

- 300 grams of button or shitake mushrooms
- 1 teaspoon olive oil
- 2 onions roughly chopped
- 3 garlic cloves
- 300 ml of chicken or vegetable stock
- 100 ml cream
- 1 pinch of Pepper or oregano powder
- Salt to taste
- Basil leaves for garnishing

Preparation

1. Thoroughly wash the mushrooms and slice them into pieces. Set aside.

2. Now take a large sized sauce pan and add 1 teaspoon of olive oil to it. Slice the garlic cloves, put them in the pan and let them simmer for a while.

3. Once the garlic turns golden brown, add the onions and sauté for about 4-5 minutes on slow heat. Now add the chopped mushrooms and fry them for another 4-5 minutes.

4. Next, add the stock to this mixture and let it boil until it the mixture softens. Add salt and pepper or oregano. Once done, let it cool down for 10-15 minutes.

5. Use an electric blender and blend the soup until it becomes smooth and has no lumps. Now transfer this mixture again onto the sauce pan and add cream to it and let it heat up for another 3-4 minutes. Switch off the gas and serve.

Serving

Instead of those boring soup bowls, you can serve this soup in large cups or deep soup plates. Garnish the soup with basil leaves. Serve this hot soup with whole-wheat or multigrain toasted garlic bread.

Variations

- You can use the same recipe using ripe pumpkin.
- Instead of cream, you can also use a bit of milk to make the soup creamy. But ensure that the use of milk is kept to a minimum.
- While roasting the garlic bread, apply some mozzarella cheese to it once in a while. Cheese when eaten in limited quantities should not cause any harm.

Recipe#14 Tofu Salad Wrap (Serves 2)

Tofu, as we all know contains substantial amount of proteins. You can either buy it from a store or make it at home. Can make Tofu at home? Indeed you can. How? We may reveal the secret recipe in our forthcoming books...

Ingredients

- 4-5 Iceberg or Romanian lettuce leaves
- 2-3 avocados
- 2 ripe tomatoes
- 1 chopped Onion + 1 for garnishing
- 1 cup Tofu
- Some Parsley
- Some salt to taste
- 1 Pinch of pepper powder
- 1 teaspoon lime juice
- 2 sheets of tortillas

Preparation

1. The first step is to mash the ripe avocadoes properly. Slice the tomatoes, onion, parsley and Romanian lettuce.

2. Now put these ingredients in a large bowl and add pieces of tofu to it. Squeeze some lime juice into it. Add salt, some pepper powder and toss it well.

3. Take tortilla sheets and place them on a tray. Now carefully fill them with the salad mixture and roll them. You can secure the roll with a toothpick.

Serving

Take a couple of lettuce leaves and place them on a large white dish, one on top of the other. Now place the tortillas on top of them and serve. You can insert a couple of olives or cherry tomatoes on the tip of the toothpick to make it look more appealing. You can serve this wrap with a yogurt and mint dip.

Variations

- If tofu is not readily available, you can fry an egg and place it on the tortillas before filling the mixture.

- One can also add a tablespoon of oats or brown rice to this salad. Try this only if your child does not mind oats.

- Fry the tortillas on a pan using a slight bit of olive oil. Once the tortilla becomes slightly crispy, add the mixture and wrap it. This will bring a bit of more crunch to the dish.

- You can also make a brown bread sandwich out of the same filling.

RECIPE #15 Yummy Salmon Salad

Salmon is an excellent, lean source of protein as well as healthy omega acids.
It is low in sodium which makes it a nice addition to the alkaline diet. My Paleo style husband loves it too. This salad is really quick to prepare, raw and high in nutrients. A recommend for Alkaline Paleo fans as well!

Serves-4

Ingredients:

- A few strips of smoked salmon, cut into smaller pieces
- Half cup of almonds
- 2 carrots, peeled (unless organic) and sliced
- 1 cucumber, peeled and sliced
- 1 onion, minced
- 2 cups of baby spinach
- 4 big tomatoes, sliced

- 2 garlic cloves, minced
- 2 big peppers, chopped
- Optional: ¼ of iceberg lettuce
- Juice of 1 lemon and olive oil
- Himalaya salt and rosemary herb

Preparation:
1. Wash all the ingredients, peel and chop.
2. Mix in a big bowl.
3. Sprinkle over some olive oil and lemon juice.
4. Add Himalaya salt to taste.
5. Enjoy, we do!

OPTIONAL: you can replace smoked salmon with chicken, sardines, or even tofu. It all depends on your family preferences. I also like to add some brown rice and chickpeas (not that alkaline, but at the same time natural and not that acidic either, this is why it is always a great choice).

Remember this simple rule:

If you want to reduce meat and are looking for more natural, vegan sources of protein, simply combine natural grains (for example brown rice, quinoa, millet) with legumes (black beans, lentils, chickpeas). The proportion should be:

Grains: Legumes- 3/1

Again, I am not telling you to go vegan, I am just providing you with some healthy options that can be also done on a budget.

RECIPE #16 Mediterranean Pasta Salad with Tuna

Another quick recipe inspired by traditional Southern European Diet. My kids love pasta and so do I. It's totally acceptable to have small amounts of integral, gluten-free pasta in your salad. Kids need energy, right?

Serves-4
Ingredients:

- About 2 cups of pasta, cooked, drained and cooled down
- Half iceberg lettuce, washed, dried and chopped
- 1 cup of baby spinach, washed, dried and chopped
- 1 big avocado, washed, peeled, pitted and chopped
- 2 cans of tuna
- 2 tomatoes, washed and sliced

- 2 carrots, washed, peeled (unless organic) and sliced
- 2 cucumbers, washed, peeled and sliced
- 1 big onion, minced
- 2 garlic cloves, peeled and minced
- Olive oil
- Juice of 2 lemons
- Optional: 2 tablespoons of soy lecithin granules (equals to better memory and concentration- great for both kids and adults)

Instructions:
1. Simply mix all the veggies and pasta in a big bowl.
2. Sprinkle over some olive oil and lemon juice.
3. Add salt to taste.
4. Enjoy!

You can store this salad in a fridge (don't add olive oil to a bowl if you want to store it, just add it when serving). I usually cook more pasta on weekend and freeze it in small containers. I do the same with rice, quinoa, lentils etc. preparation is the key and I always make sure I have some food ready or almost ready to grab.

VARIATIONS:
Instead of pasta you can use brown rice, millet, and amaranth and basmati rice.
You can also spice it up with some nice, raw salsa. I usually blend avocados with some coconut milk, lemon juice and chilli. It has a nice and creamy consistency that is also a bit spicy. Add to it some garlic and you have a super healthy, natural salsa that will get your kids hooked on salads and veggies! Colors can help.

RECIPE #17 Apple and Veggie Salad

This recipe is all about being creative.

I work as a Spanish teacher and I very often work with little children. When learning new words, for example verbs, I usually ask them in Spanish:

"What can you do with an apple? What can you do with a carrot? Can you eat it? Can you cut it?"

..."And how about adding some spinach?"

Children are much more creative than adults. They also soak languages like a sponge! The same rule applies to healthy eating. So don't wait till tomorrow. Get your kids started now. Encourage creativity. It will also be fun for you!

Ask your children: "Can you eat apples in a salad?"

See what they say and play with it. If they say: "Yes", tell them: "Why, how did you know? Do you know how to make an apple salad? Because I don't know! Help me!".

If, on the other hand, they say: "No, you can't", ask them: "Hmm...hold on a second. The other day I was at my friend's house and she made an apple salad. She said you could do it too. So please tell me how to do it! I REALLY wanna know".

Let's keep playing!

Serves-4
Ingredients:
- 2 big apples, peeled, pitted and chopped
- 1 avocado, peeled, pitted and chopped
- 2 tomatoes, slices
- 2 carrots, peeled and sliced
- 1 big pepper (green, red or orange), sliced

- Juice of 1 lemon
- Olive oil
- Himalaya Salt
- 1 cup of green olives, pitted
- A few raisins

Instructions:
1. Mix all the ingredients in a bowl.
2. Add olive oil, lemon juice and Himalaya salt.
3. Don't forget about olives and raisins! An excellent combination!

RECIPE #18 Chicken Soup

We love this recipe in the winter. Chicken and veggies are excellent combination and totally compatible with both Alkaline and Paleo lifestyle.

Serves-4

Soup:

- 2 liter chicken broth
- ½ lb. shredded cooked chicken (leftovers work well)
- 1 large rib celery, dice or chop
- 2 carrots, dice or chop
- 1 onion
- 4 garlic cloves
- 1 cup of mushrooms
- 2 zucchini, use a grater, peeler or slicer to make noodles
- Salt/pepper to taste (if you like crushed red pepper or cayenne please add)

Instructions:

1. Boil the broth and add the cooked chicken. Turn to low and simmer.

2. Put in the carrots, mushrooms, onion, garlic cloves and celery for 20 min.

3. Now, add zucchini noodles and cook 3-4 min longer.

RECIPE #19 VEGGIE STRI-FRY WITH COLORS!

This recipe is all about colors!

Serves-4

Ingredients:

- A few slices of tofu (can be also fish, chicken or even bacon, it's up to you!)
- 1 big onion, peeled and minced
- 2 garlic cloves, peeled and minced
- Coconut oil
- A few tablespoons of coconut milk
- A few big peppers (green, red and yellow), I usually go for 6 big peppers of mixed colors
- 2 zucchini
- Himalaya Salt

Preparation:

1. In a saucepan, heat up a few tablespoons of coconut oil.

2. Add garlic and onions and stir for a few minutes.
3. Add tofu. Stir-fry until brownish.
4. Add salt and a bit of coconut milk. Lower the heat.
5. Add chopped veggies and stir-fry until soft (low heat, 15 minutes).
6. Serve with a few lime or lemon slices.
7. Enjoy!

RECIPE #20 ALKALINE VEGETERIAN CURRY

We adore Asian cooking and spices. This is a really simplified version of vegetarian curry that is really easy and quick to prepare. Kids love it!

Serves-4
Ingredients:

- 4 cups of basmati rice, cooked (as per instructions)
- 1 cup of chickpeas (boiled, you can also get canned chickpeas if you are pressed for time)
- 4 big carrots, peeled, halved and sliced (really thin!)
- 2 big zucchini, peeled and sliced (as thin as possible!)
- 1 onion, cut in rings

- A few teaspoons of curry powder
- Himalaya salt to taste
- Coconut oil
- Coconut milk
- Lime

Preparation:
1. Fry onion in coconut oil until brownish.
2. Reduce the heat, add coconut milk (half cup) and veggies. Add curry powder to taste (a few teaspoons)
3. Stir-fry until soft. If necessary add more coconut milk or oil.
4. Add rice and chickpeas. Stir energetically.
5. Add salt, pepper and more curry if necessary.
6. Sprinkle over some lime juice.
7. We like to accompany this dish with some green, alkaline juice (for example apple and spinach).
8. Enjoy!

RECIPE #21 SUNDAY VEGGIE ROAST COMPETITION!

Another creative dish. All you need is lots of different veggies, spices, coconut oil and if you wish you can also use some bacon and cheese. Tofu is also great for that if you want to make it more alkaline.

This is what we made last Sunday. We all participated and had fun!

Serves-4
Ingredients:
- 4 big potatoes, sliced
- 2 cups of broccoli crowns, chopped
- Oregano, rosemary and basil
- Olive oil
- Himalaya salt
- 2 big tomatoes, sliced
- 4 carrots

- 4 zucchini
- A few strips of bacon
- 1 onion, cut in rings

Preparation:
1. Mix all the veggies with herbs, salt and spices. Add bacon if you wish. Place in a big baking mold.
2. Add some olive oil and mix.
3. Bake for about 1 h (180 Celsius).

RECIPE #22 Carrots Aperitif for Big Boys!

This is a fantastic alkaline aperitif!

Serves-2 big boys

Ingredients:

- 3, 4 carrots, (cut in smaller sticks)
- 1 cucumber
- 1 avocado
- 2 tomatoes
- 2 tablespoons of coconut oil
- Himalaya salt

Preparation:

1. Blend avocado + tomatoes + cucumber.
2. Add some coconut oil and mix.
3. Add salt and pepper to taste.
4. Serve with carrot sticks. Cucumber sticks or radishes are also great.

5. Enjoy, we love this quick recipe when awaiting our main dish! Big boys are always hungry, right?

RECIPE #23 Veggie Pizza

Kids love pizza. It's up to you, if you want to make it healthy.

Spices, cheese and veggies are such a great combination. Here comes a super healthy comfort food recipe!

Serves-4

Ingredients:
- 4 big zucchini, sliced (very thin)
- 4 tomatoes
- 2 onions
- ¼ cup of parmesan cheese or goats cheese (grated or in slices)

- 2 big peppers, sliced
- 2 cups of mushrooms, sliced
- Olive oil
- Salt, oregano, rosemary and basil.

Preparation:
1. Preheat the oven to 180 degrees.
2. Smear your usual pizza mold with some olive oil.
3. Place zucchini slices first.
4. Add the rest of veggies and slices on top.
5. Sprinkle over some parmesan cheese.
6. Bake for about 30 minutes.
7. Enjoy! So yummy!

Chapter 3: Alkaline Dinners/Snacks and Afternoon Meals

The best part about enjoying an alkaline dinner is that you can even afford to overeat a bit. An alkaline meal may seem like there's a lot on the plate, yet you won't feel overstuffed. This also helps in eliminating those post dinner cravings, where the children end up snacking on unhealthy fried food like chips or cheese balls.

RECIPE #24 Steamed fish in mint paste and lemon (Serves 2 or 3)

Most people debate about the acidic nature of fish. The fact is that fish is very mildly acidic in nature. Hence, it can be consumed in moderation. When you combine fish with mint or lemon, the alkalinity of these two items takes over the slightly acidic properties of fish and provides you with a well balanced dish.

Ingredients

- 450 grams of fish fillet
- 2 tablespoons of olive oil
- Ginger garlic paste
- 2 lemons (1 for the recipe+1 for garnishing)
- 1 Pinch of pepper powder
- 1 green chilli
- 1 cup of mint leaves
- ½ cup of coriander leaves
- Approximately 1 teaspoon of salt (as per taste)
- 1 pinch of turmeric
- 50 ml water

Preparation

1. Place the fish fillet in a large bowl and set them aside.

2. Firstly, we need to prepare the mint paste. For this, take the mint leaves, coriander leaves,

and green chilli and put it in the grinder. Add a bit of salt, water and grind this mixture until it turns slightly smoother. This mint paste is always coarsely grounded and will not have a paste like consistency.

3. Now mix the mint paste, ginger garlic paste, turmeric, some salt and apply it to the fish fillets in the bowl. Cover the fish fillets fully with this paste, Squeeze a lemon on top of them and keep it in the fridge for about 30 minutes for marinating.

4. Remove the bowl from the fridge. Now pack these fish one at a time using a paper foil and keep them aside.

5. Steam the fish for about 10 minutes and switch off the flame.

Serving

You can serve the fish on a banana leaf to give it a nice tropical feel. You can also use an entire fish without slicing it. This makes the dish look more interesting than it already is. Just let it marinate for a few more minutes, so the mixture is properly absorbed by fish. Cut ultra-thin slices of lemons and place them on the fish or on the edges of the banana leaf.

Variations:

- You can use the same marinating process for cottage cheese instead of fish.
- For steaming, wrap the marinated fish into a banana or jackfruit leaf. It will bring a nice flavor to the dish.

Recipe #25 Whole Wheat Pasta with Tomatoes, Broccoli and Almonds (Serves 2)

This nutritious pasta easily scores over the fattening macaroni and cheese.

Ingredients

- 200 gms of whole wheat pasta
- 7-8 almonds
- 1 bowls of broccoli (200 gms)
- 1 chopped tomato
- Olive or coconut oil
- 3-4 garlic cloves
- 1 or 2 green chillies
- 1 tablespoon salt
- 1 teaspoon of pepper powder
- Basil leaves for garnishing

Preparation

1. Take a large vessel, fill it with water and let it boil. Once it reaches the boiling point, throw in the pasta and cook it until it becomes

tender. When the pasta starts to feel softer, drain the water. Add half of a teaspoon of olive oil to the pasta and mix it well. This will prevent the pasta from sticking.

2. Cut the broccoli into small pieces and blanch them for about 2 minutes in hot water.

3. Take a saucepan and place it on slow heat. Add oil and almonds to it and sauté them until they turn bright brown in color. Remember you want the almonds to be crunchy. Now add the chopped tomatoes to this mixture and cook until they are mushy.

4. Cut the garlic cloves, green chillies in thin slices and add them into the pan. Fry the garlic until its light brown. Next, add the blanched broccoli and let it simmer until it becomes softer.

5. As soon as you notice that the broccoli has gotten tender, put in the pasta. Add some salt and toss it well.

Serving

Always serve the pasta in a big bowl. It's easier to eat for the kids without them spilling. Garnish the pasta with leaves on top. You can also slice up a green capsicum and insert a strand in the centre.

Variation

- Whole wheat noodles can be used in place of pasta.
- Broccoli can be replaced with any other alkaline vegetable your kid is fond of.
- You can always add olive or use any other dry fruits other than almonds.

Recipe #26 Rose flavored Soy Milk Pudding with Roasted almonds on top (Serves 2)

All kids adore deserts. Here's a healthy desert your kid can enjoy without consuming too many calories. What's more, it's nutritious too.

Ingredients

- 450 ml rice milk
- 3 tablespoons corn starch
- 2 or 3 tablespoons of brown sugar
- 2 drops of rose concentrate
- 1 egg
- 7-8 almonds

Preparation

1. Take a large bowl with corn starch in it and slowly add the milk. Keep stirring it so it does not form any lumps.

2. Now crack an egg into this mixture, add brown sugar and stir again properly. Add two or three drops of rose concentrate to it and cook the mixture on a medium heat. Cover it with a lid until it cooks for about 15-20 minutes.

3. Slice the almonds into two halves and roast them on a flat pan on medium heat. Spread the roasted almonds on top of the pudding.

Serving

If you can get your hand on those small earthen pots, you can fill them with the pudding and refrigerate it for 30 minutes. This chilled pudding will be a perfect desert without having to worry about your child putting on too much weight. This dessert can also be served in fancy glass bowls.

Variations

- Rice milk has high nutritional properties but so does oats milk / soy (GMO free) milk and hazelnut milk. Try it and choose your favorite taste or combination of tastes.

- Instead of using corn starch and eggs for the pudding, you can dissolve 2-2/12 teaspoon of gelatin in the milk to get that perfect jelly-like formation.

- Roasted almonds can be replaced with dry figs or even pistachios.

- Just like rose concentrate, vanilla or strawberry flavor goes very well with this pudding.

- If you wish to try a variation with this pudding, add a bit of melted dark chocolate while using the same type of preparation. The rest of the ingredients would be the same. All you need to do is infuse some dark chocolate. You may want to go easy with additional sugar as dark chocolate brings its own sweetness to this dish.

It is very essential for children to eat at least four meals a day. This can help in maintaining their body's metabolic rate as well. If your child is obese, there is an all the more reason to make him/her eat all four meals a day. Obesity isn't always caused by over eating. It is a result of erratic eating schedules combined with the wrong foodstuffs.

Recipe #27 Capsicum and Corn Sandwich with Avocado Spread (Serves 2)

This *yummylicious* spread can be used instead of mayonnaise in practically every single sandwich or wraps.

Ingredients

- 1 large sized bell peppers or two small sized different color bell peppers
- One whole sweet corn (100 gms)
- 1 onion
- 1 avocado
- Coriander sprigs
- 1 green chilly
- 1 teaspoon of salt
- ½ teaspoon pepper powder
- 4 slices to brown or whole wheat bread

Preparation

1. Slice the bell peppers, onion and place them in a large vessel. Immerse the sweet corns into a boiling pot of water and drain them after about 5 minutes until the corns become slightly tender.
2. Now add all the other ingredients like salt, pepper powder and corns to the bell peppers and onions. Mix it together.
3. For the avocado spread, mash the avocados slightly and put them into the grinder. Add a few cilantro leaves, half a chilly, salt and grind the mixture until forms a paste.
4. Take the bread slices and apply the avocado spread on one of the slices. Fill the corn and bell pepper mixture to it and cover it with another bread slice.

Serving

Use a toothpick to hold the sandwich together. This yummy treat can be easily wrapped in a foil and you can carry it in the bag in case your kid is out on a picnic or an adventure trip. This sandwich will taste much better if your grill or roast it.

Variations

- Based on a similar preparation like that of the avocado spread, you can make a mint spread too.
- To avoid the monotony of serving a sandwich, you can fill this mixture inside a whole wheat croissant or turn it into a burrito.
- In order to add a bit of crunch to the sandwich filling, deep-fry some parsley and lay it on top of the mixture.

Recipe #28 Spinach and Cottage Cheese Burger (Serves 2)

We understand that burgers are your kid's favorite snack and this can be highly annoying for a parent as you know they only add to your child's weight issues. But a spinach and cottage cheese burger will certainly make you and your kid happy.

- 10-15 spinach leaves
- 200 grams of cottage cheese
- 1 or 2 green chillies
- 1 tablespoon paprika powder
- 1 tablespoon lemon juice
- Whole wheat bread crumbs
- One teaspoon salt
- 3-4 garlic cloves
- 2-3 table spoons of olive oil
- Whole wheat buns
- 2 or 3 leaves of iceberg or Romanian lettuce

Preparation

1. Crumble the cottage cheese in a bowl and set aside. Slightly blanch the spinach leaves. Later chop them and add to the crumbles cottage cheese.
2. Chop the green chillies and garlic cloves into thin slices. Add the chopped chillies, garlic, paprika powder, salt, lemon juice to the cottage cheese and mix together properly.
3. Make small sized patties using your hands, apply a bit of olive oil on them, dip them into the bread crumbs and set them on a baking tray.
4. Preheat the oven for about 5 minutes. Now bake the spinach and cottage cheese patties in the oven at 160 c for approximately 20-25 minutes until they form a nice crust on top.

Serving

Cut the whole wheat burger buns and place the patties on top of it. Now keep a lettuce leaf on top of it. Use a toothpick to bind the burger and keep it from falling apart. Insert a sliced olive on the tip of the toothpick.

Variation

- Tofu could also be used instead of cottage cheese.
- You can occasionally shallow fry the patties on a pan to save on time.
- Instead of bread crumbs, you can use semolina to coat the patties.
- Fresh cherries on the tip of the toothpick can also make the dish look attractive.

Recipe #29 Quinoa and Coriander Stuffed Tomatoes (Serves 2 or 3)

Did you say your kid does not like tomatoes? Try these stuffed tomatoes and you will never be able to say that again.

Ingredients

- 3 large sized tomatoes
- 2 Bell Peppers
- 3 or 4 Garlic Cloves
- 1 big sized Onion
- 100 gms of boiled brown or plain rice
- 6 to 7 Almonds
- 3 tablespoon extra virgin olive oil
- ½ a bowl of quinoa
- 1 ½ teaspoon salt
- 1 teaspoon paprika powder

Preparation

1. Slice the tomatoes into two and scoop the seeds and pulp out. Be careful while doing this as we need the tomato skin to remain intact.

2. Dip the quinoa into large pot of boiling water for about 4-5 minutes. Now drain out the excess water and transfer the quinoa into a bowl.

3. Thinly chop the bell peppers, almonds, garlic cloves and tomatoes and add them to the quinoa. Add these chopped ingredients to the quinoa, sprinkle some salt and paprika powder. Drizzle this mixture with extra virgin olive oil and stuff it gently into the tomatoes.

4. Place the stuffed tomatoes on a baking tray and transfer it into a preheated oven up to 180C. Bake for about 12-14 minutes at 160C. Once the tomatoes are fully baked, take them

out from the oven and let them sit for a few minutes.

Serving

On a flat dish, place some banana or cabbage leaves and gently place the tomatoes on them. Serve them slightly hot.

Variations

- Avocadoes or even stuffed bell peppers would taste just as nice as the tomatoes.
- You can use oats instead of rice.
- The stuffed tomatoes can also be cooked in a sauce pan for 15-20 minutes on medium heat by covering it with a lid.

Recipe #30 Sweet Carrot Puree

Carrots are naturally sweet, but very few people realize it.

This recipe is sweet, tasty, healthy and cheap as well! Healthy eating on a budget!

Serves-2

Ingredients:

- 4 carrots, peeled and chopped
- 2 tablespoons of honey
- Pinch of cinnamon
- 1 banana
- 1 tablespoon of coconut oil
- Half cup of almond milk

Instructions:

1. Boil carrots until soft.
2. Drain and cool down.
3. In a blender, mix with almond milk, honey, banana and coconut oil.
4. Blend until smooth.

5. Serve with a few blueberries on top.

Recipe #31 Sweet Apple and Cinnamon Drink

This is a really delicious and healthy recipe that I learned from a Polish friend of mine. It is called "compott" in Polish. My boys love it There are no sodas in our house. At first, our boys were complaining but now it's their friends who visit our house to try our original recipes and our healthy way of life!

You can have this drink warm or nicely chilled.

Ingredients for 4 serves (4 cups):
- 4 big apples, peeled and chopped

- 2 teaspoons of cinnamon powder
- 1 cup of strawberries
- 1 liter of water
- 2 tablespoons of honey
- 1 teaspoon of vanilla extract

Instructions:

1. Put water to boil.
2. Turn off the heat when boiling.
3. Add apples and strawberries. Sweeten with honey and vanilla.
4. Cover and leave for a few hours.
5. Serve with a few leaves of fresh mint!

Recipe #32 Orange-Choco Smoothie

Orange juice is a great source of natural vitamin C and so are the lemons. But how to make our kids love it? It's simple: choco it up!

Serves-2

Ingredients:

- Fresh juice of 2 oranges
- Half cup of water
- Juice of 1 lemon
- 1 cup of almond milk
- 2-3 tablespoons of raw cocoa powder!
- Half banana

Preparation:
1. Blend all ingredients in a blender.
2. Serve with some creative ice cubes (like frozen juice) or frozen blueberries.
3. Enjoy!

Recipe #33 Roibosh Banana Smoothie

Roibosh is a natural caffeine-free infusion that has a nice, sweet taste. It is a great source of antioxidants as well.

I like to use it as a base for nutritious smoothies. So much better than plain water!

Serves-2

Ingredients:

- 1 cup of roibosh tea, cooled
- 2 bananas, peeled and chopped
- 1 avocado, peeled, pitted and chopped
- A bit of cinnamon, stevia or honey to sweeten
- Half cup of coconut milk

Preparation

1. Mix all the ingredients in a blender.

2. Serve with a few ice cubes. Sprinkle over some raw cocoa powder on top. I also like to add a few raisins or almond powder.

Recipe #34 Mediterranean Fruit Salad

This is an excellent snack recipe!

Serves-2

Ingredients:
- 1 cup of cooked couscous
- 1 grapefruit, peeled and sliced
- 1 orange, peeled and sliced
- 1 kiwi, peeled and sliced
- ½ cup of blueberries
- 2 tablespoons of honey mixed with coconut milk
- A few raisins and almonds

Instructions:
1. In a bowl, mix couscous with fruits.

2. Add raisins, almonds, honey and coconut milk.
3. Optional: sprinkle over some lime juice and cinnamon.
4. So yummy and healthy!

Recipe #35 Alkaline Spanish Granizado

Granizado is a juice that is almost frozen. Great alkaline recipe for hot summers!

Serves- 2 cups
Ingredients:
- 1 cup of almond milk
- 1 cup of fresh grapefruit and lemon juice
- ½ cup of blueberries or strawberry slices

Instructions:
1. Mix all the ingredients (one big cup or 2 separate ones).
2. Place in a fridge for about 40 minutes. We don't want it 100% frozen, just some part of it.
3. Serve with a few raisins on top!
4. Enjoy! So alkaline and delicious!

Recipe #36 Apple-Kiwi Marmalade

My boys love this recipe with fruits or toasts.

Serves-2

Ingredients:
- 2 kiwis, peeled and sliced
- 2 ripe apples, peeled and sliced
- A few pineapple slices (optional)
- Coconut oil
- Cinnamon Powder/stevia
- A few tablespoons of coconut milk

Instructions:
1. Blend all the ingredients (add coconut milk)
2. Fry slightly in coconut oil for about 5 minutes /low heat/.
3. Add a bit of cinnamon and stevia to sweeten.
4. Cool down in a fridge.

5. Serve with fresh fruits, ice-cream, toasts, oat meals…
6. Enjoy, we love it!

Recipe #37 Wakame Energy Smoothie Made Sweet

Wakame is an alg that, even though does not taste super delicious, is an excellent source of Calcium, Magnesium, Iron and Phosphorus. I mastered the art of smoothies and my kids consume wakame daily, without even knowing what it is!

Serves- 2 cups
Ingredients:
- 1 banana, peeled and sliced
- 2 peaches, peeled, pitted and sliced
- 1 avocado, peeled, pitted and sliced
- 2 cups of almond milk
- Juice of 1 lemon

- A few dates, pitted
- About 5 square inches of alga wakame

Instructions:
1. Soak wakame in filtered water for about 15 mins.
2. Once wakame is soft, blend with the rest of ingredients until smooth.
3. Sprinkle over some raw cocoa powder! Health is tasty!

Recipe #38 COCO Dream

This is an excellent exotic style smoothie!

Serves- 2

Ingredients:
- 1 cup of coconut milk
- 1 cup of coconut water
- A few pineapple slices
- A few watermelon slices
- A few mango slices

Instructions:
1. Mix all the ingredients in a blender.
2. Serve immediately with a few lemon/lime slices and ice cubes.
3. Enjoy!

Recipe #39 Delicious Apple Tortillas

Another fruity- juicy and tasty recipe!

Serves-2

Ingredients:

- 2 free range eggs
- 2 apples, peeled and grated
- 2 teaspoons of vanilla extract
- 4 tablespoons of almond powder
- Coconut oil

Instructions:

1. Mix/ blend all the ingredients until smooth.
2. Heat coconut oil in a frying pan.
3. Form 2 little tortillas and fry.
4. Serve with alkaline fruity marmalade from previous recipes.

Recipe #40 Kale and Spinach Chips

This is an excellent natural, alkaline snack!

Serves-a few cups

Ingredients:

- A few cups of mixed kale and spinach leaves
- Mix of different spices and salt
- Coconut oil

Instructions:

1. Preheat the oven (180 degrees).
2. In the meantime, "massage" kale and spinach leaves in coconut oil. Make sure all the leaves are equally "massaged" and "nourished".
3. Place spinach and kale in the oven, sprinkle over some salt and spices.
4. Bake for about 30 minutes.
5. We love this snack with guacamole!

Recipe #41 Beet and Orange Magic!

Are your kids thirsty after playing around on a hot afternoon?

Serves- 4 cups

Ingredients:

For the beet ice cubes:

- 1 cup of beet and almond milk smoothie frozen into ice cubes
- 1 cup of frozen blueberries
- 1 liter of water
- A few slices of lime and lemon
- Stevia to sweeten

Instructions:

Simply mix all the ingredients in a jar! Ice cubes will do an amazing effect when melting!

Additional Tips:

1. Water- hydration is really important. Use your imagination and prepare fresh fruit infused water every day. Freeze fruits and fruit juices so that they serve you as amazingly creative ice cubes that are fun with all their colors and tastes.
2. Use all kinds of caffeine free teas and herbal infusions that your whole family can benefit from:
    - Rosemary
    - Thyme (both are great to stimulate the immune system)
    - Ginger (will also help keep your family strong and healthy)
    - Mint and chamomile (for better sleep and improved digestion).

3. Use cooled herbal infusions for natural ice teas and infuse them with fruits and herbs.

Your imagination is the only limit to what can be achieved!

Conclusion

Alkaline meals are not only lighter on the stomach but they also leave you feeling fuller and energized throughout the day. Kids need a lot of energy between going to school, playing, studying and extracurricular activities. Getting your kid to eat healthy alkaline food may seem pretty impossible at the start. But if you make your meals more fun and innovative, the kids will fall in love with it without knowing that they are actually eating the same healthy food which they once thought is as 'sad.' When you are dealing with your kids, innovation is the key. They just can't imagine themselves eating the same food every day.

While most kids demand a burger or chocolate tarts while coming back home from school, our interesting alkaline dishes will make them look forward to home cooked meals. Do not refuse them their daily snack of fries right away. Instead, tell your child that he/she can have whatever they want but there is a surprise meal waiting for them at home. This will give rise to their curiosity and gradually discourage them from eating all kinds of "forbidden fruits".

If you pass on healthy eating habits to your children at an early age, it will be easier for them to make it a part of their lifestyle. The recipes given in this book will help you entice your kid into eating alkaline food which will eventually even cure their obesity problems if any. I have presented you with more than 40 different and innovative recipes with step by step explanation of the preparation process. Each recipe has a new twist to it.

Now it's your turn! I am sure that your kids will love it!

Finally, if you enjoyed this book and you have a few seconds, please rank it on Amazon and post your honest review. It's you I am writing for, and I love hearing from my readers.

HOW TO LEAVE A REVIEW?

1. LOG INTO YOUR ACCOUNT

2. GO TO THIS LINK:
   http://www.amazon.com/dp/B00MQ8YVZO

3. If you use Amazon UK, go to:
   http://www.amazon.co.uk/dp/B00MQ8YVZO

4. If you use Amazon Canada, go to:
   http://www.amazon.ca/dp/B00MQ8YVZO

5. If you use Amazon Australia, go to:
   http://www.amazon.com.au/dp/B00MQ8YVZO

6. Simply click on "Customers Reviews".

7. Go to "Create Your Own Review".

8. Select the ranking (1-5 stars, of course I am always more than happy with positive rankings, however I can also receive critical feedback).

9. Share your thoughts on my book. Even 2 words will do!

If you have any questions, suggestions or feedback, you can also reach me via e-mail:

Elenajamesbooks@gmail.com

I hope to "see" you in my new books!

I also suggest you follow this facebook/twitter page:

www.facebook.com/HolisticWellnessBooks

www.twitter.com/Wellness_Books

If you like free and $0.99 books and kindle countdowns, Holistic Wellness Books is a place for you to "hang out"!

I have created it with a few fellow authors that also write books on health, fitness and personal development.

Thanks in advance for taking interest in our work!

I wish you energy, health and success!

Elena Garcia

www.facebook.com/HolisticWellnessBooks

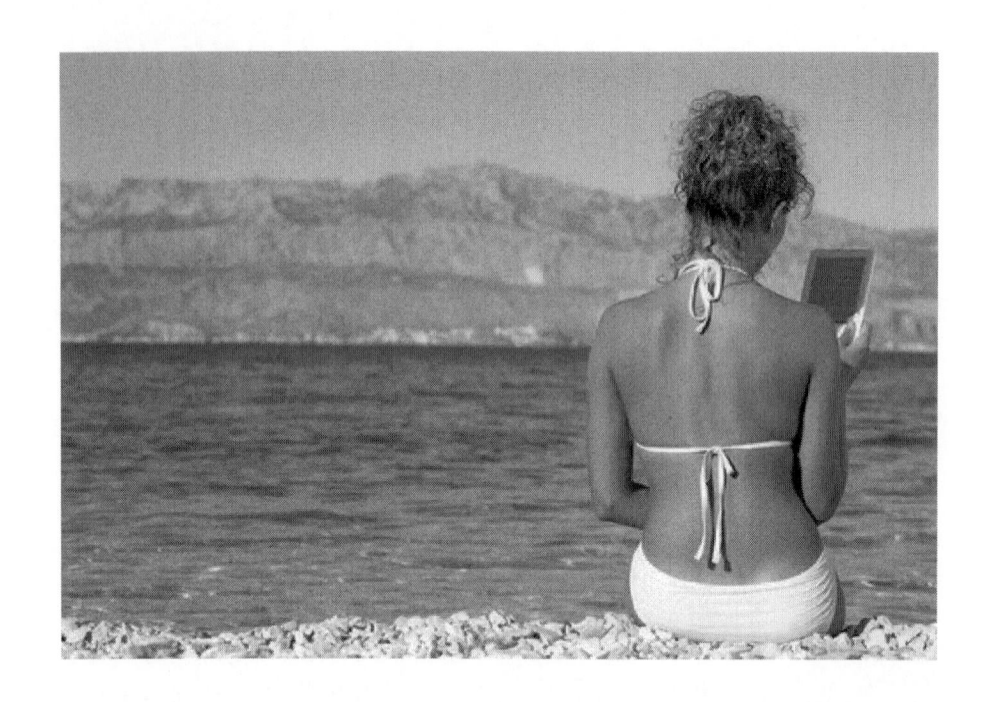

MORE BOOKS BY ELENA GARCIA AND HER HUSBAND:

Alkaline Weight Loss and Wellness

The Mediterranean Diet Rocks!

Alkaline Paleo Recipes

Ayurveda Rocks!

The Paleo Diet for Weight Loss and Health

NLP for Weight Loss

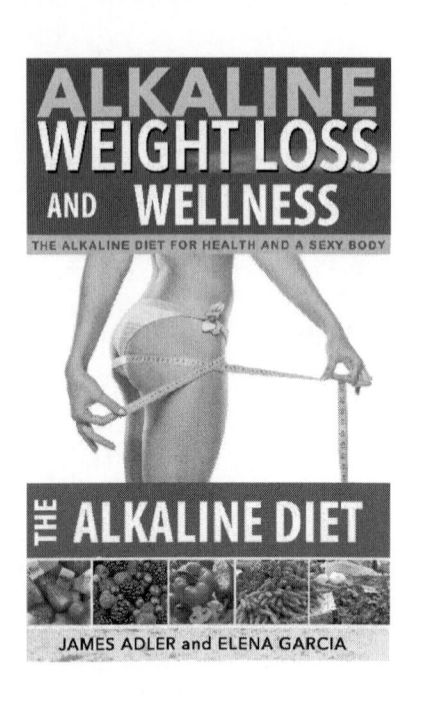

Recommended reading by other authors:

Gluten-free, recipes, healthy lifestyle, weight loss series by Annette Goodman

Smoothies for Holistic Wellness and Weight Loss by Marta Tuchowska

Fruit Infused Spa Water by Marta Tuchowska

Healthy Eating on a Budget by Dexter Poin

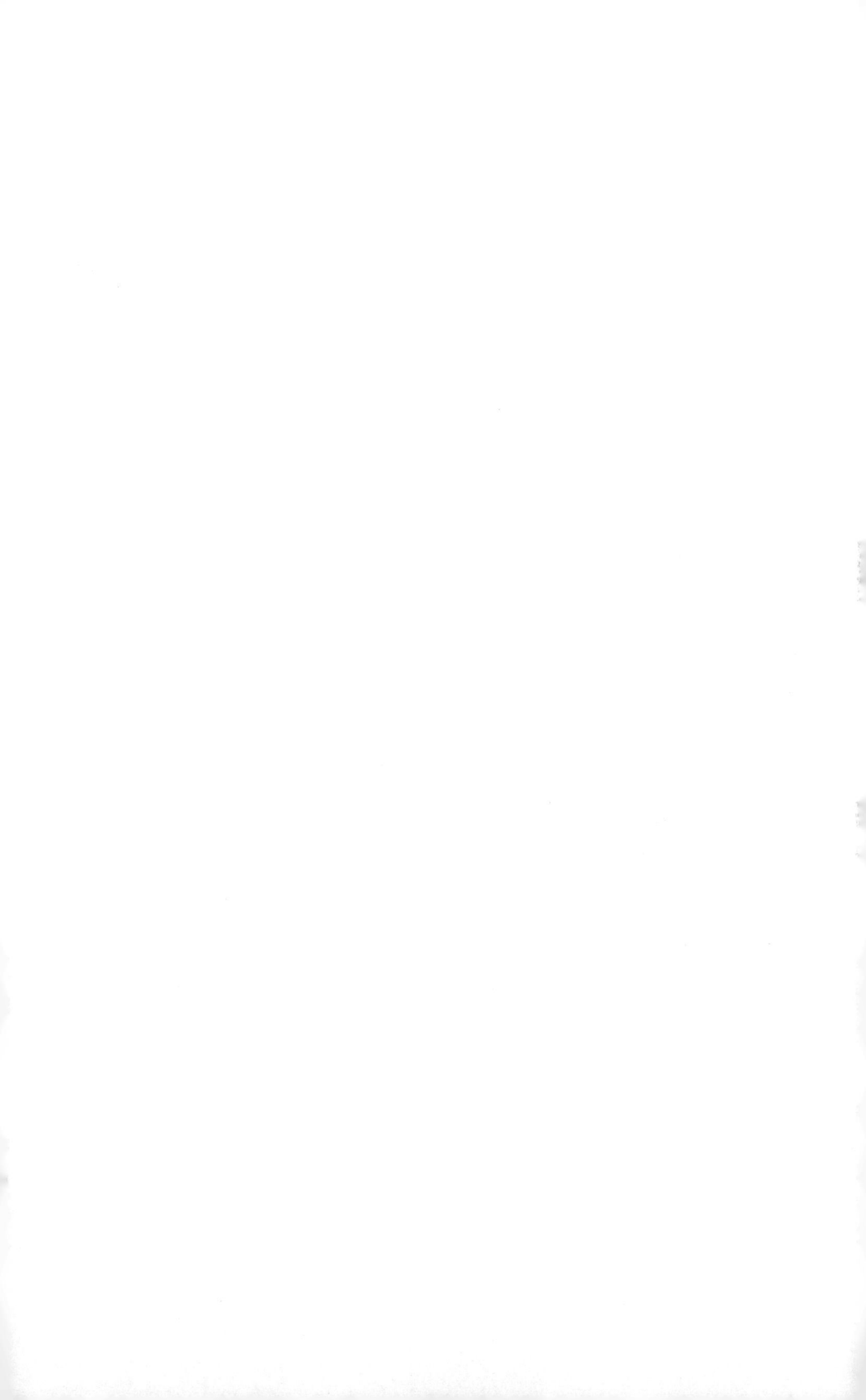

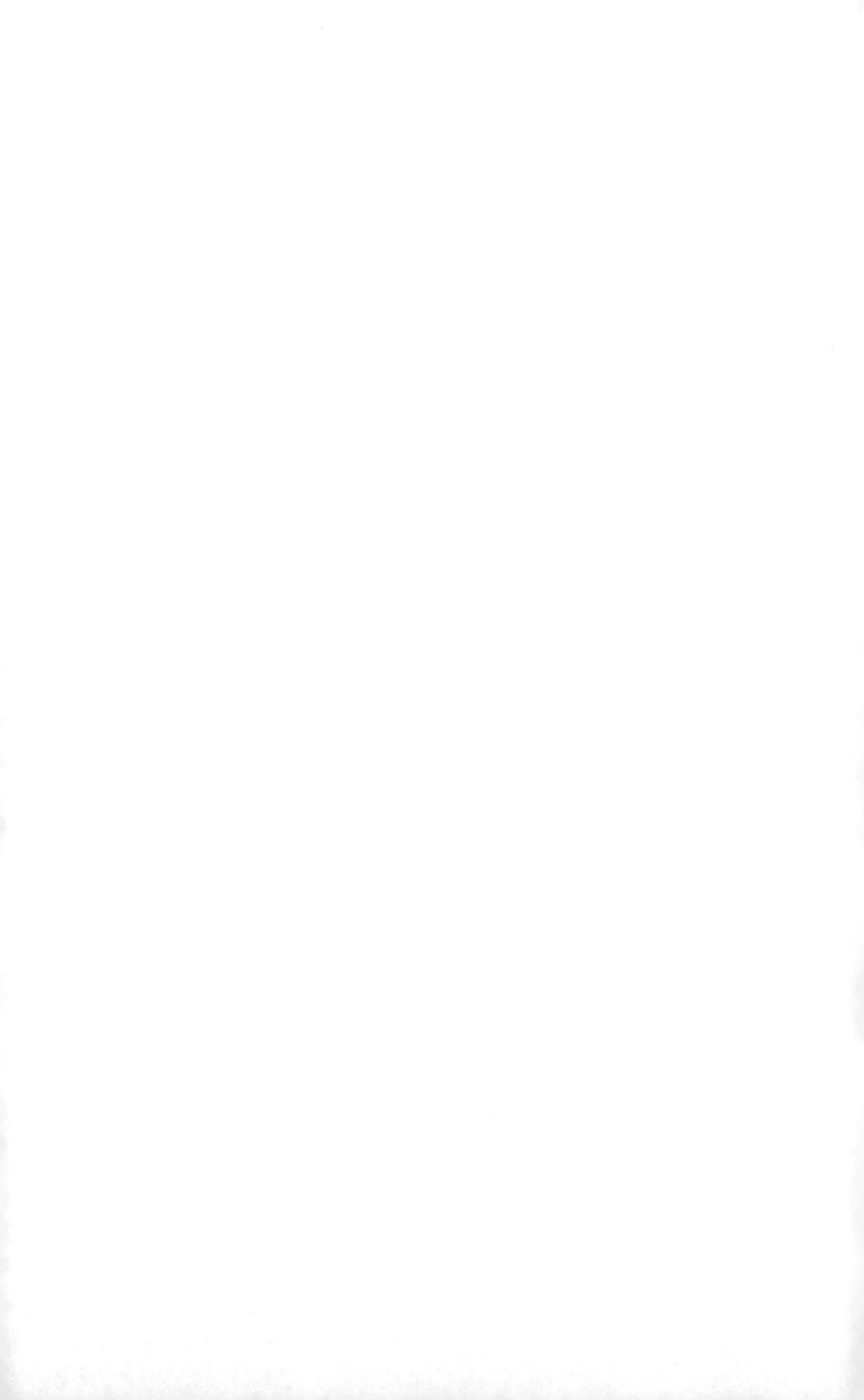

Printed in Great Britain
by Amazon.co.uk, Ltd.,
Marston Gate.